JOY JOY VAN

Walk Your Weight Down

The easiest (and perhaps most humorous) way to shed pounds while boosting your well being

*To the Fab 5 - you know who you are - and of course Earl -thanks for bringing
me so much happiness!*

"Walking is man's best medicine."

-Hippocrates

Contents

I

Part One

1

The introduction you never asked for…..

Welcome to Walk Your Weight Down, the easiest way to shed some weight we carry around infused with a sprinkle of humor (I gave it my best shot). I would like to extend my heartfelt thanks to you for picking up this book even if you really didn't want to.

My name is Joy (many call me Joy Joy or even Joyous) and I have worked in the fitness industry for over 15+ years. I have taught a variety of exercise modalities and have worked with clients ranging from ages 13-90. I have even made a few nutritional, knock-out smoothies for many individuals to help them reach some personal dietary goals at one of my favorite fuel bars in a club where I was teaching fitness classes. With that being said, I do have a genuine desire to help others set and achieve realistic health and wellness goals which is why I chose to write this book. Also, I love social interaction and have often been perceived as a person who is an optimist living in a state of constant rays of sunshine (this can totally be refuted by my hubby FYI). If you can't relate to that - well, clearly we can't be friends but this book is not about me becoming your buddy. In fact, you really do NOT have to like me at all. My name alone can be offensive to some and I get it. I have been called naive, gullible and even fake and I am actually OK with all of it.

This book is not about me. It is about you taking the first step towards the betterment of your life by incorporating walking as a form of letting some weight go and finding a little bit of happiness along the way. Will everyday be filled with rainbows and lollipops after reading this book? Probably not, but my hope for you is that you can find a way to make some small changes that do bring a little more joy into your life - pun intended.

So why wait? Let's get started!

2

It's you, hello, you're the problem, it's you…..

Wow! You thought this book was going to be funny, motivational and filled with positivity but before we really get into the exciting parts, we have to look in the mirror and face some harsh truths. I recently attended a training course where I had to take a real look, not just a side eye glance, a real big looky-loo at myself and man I was gobsmacked. The real truth of the matter is we are products of the decisions we have made that have led us to this very moment in our lives. We can no longer blame things or people for where we are right now. For example, how many times have you projected your individual shortcomings or misfortunes on to other people or circumstances in order to protect your own insecurities? I know I have. We live in a world of "if only I had this, I could be this" or "if my parents had done this, I would have been so much better off" but I am here to tell you that stops now. Say this 5 times out loud - "It's me, hello, I'm the problem, it's me!" Dang - sounds like a catchy tune doesn't it?

Why the heck am I talking about this? I have heard every possible excuse and explanation as to why people are unhappy when it comes to their physical and emotional well being. I am an empathetic person - don't get me wrong but at some point, I stop listening when I see no effort in making a change. In other words, lip service is out of business today! If you can stop the blame game by confronting yourself at this very given moment, you will begin to make the biggest transformation of your life. I encourage you to take a minute to get curious about what is holding you back in relation to your physical and emotional well being. Check in with yourself daily and don't be afraid to ask "what am I noticing about myself today?" especially when things seem to be going down the loo. Focus on YOU and your own decisions and choose NOT to blame things such as gender, race, parents, living conditions, economic status, class, education etc...When you begin to shift your focus towards who you are today and who you want to be tomorrow, you will begin to unburden yourself from any weight that you are carrying around and change the way you live.

3

Why excuses stink and the best ones out there…..

One of my mom's favorite sayings will forever be ingrained in my brain - "fish and company start to smell after three days." I laugh (and kind of cringe) every time she says it and I think the same goes for when I hear people making excuses for their behavior. They start to STINK! Let's debunk some popular excuses for getting out of walking down the weight.

I just don't have time….

I literally can't even deal with this excuse. Let's take the President of the United States (this will not be about politics I promise!) We have seen presidents out running, biking, riding horses, swimming and playing golf. Regardless of how you feel about the president, I would imagine he/she has a pretty stressful and jam packed schedule yet still finds some time for some healthy habits.

It ultimately once again comes down to YOU. What are your priorities? Could you wake up earlier, sneak a walk in during your lunch break or incorporate some walking into your day/days off? How about even parking in the farthest spot away from the entrance at the grocery store? When my daughters were little, I spent hours in the car as a "m-uber driver" (Mom Uber and I just made that up). I would always keep a pair of walking shoes in the vehicle for when I had a few extra minutes while waiting for them to finish up a school or sport related activity. Did I look crazy walking around the middle school parking lot? Probably but I sure felt better afterwards. Take inventory of your daily routine and be honest. Remember - the most dangerous lies can be the ones we tell ourselves. (Good one right?) How much time are you using up watching TV or scrolling through social media? Could you initially carve out just an extra 10/15 minutes in your day? If getting alone time is nearly impossible, I encourage you to start inside your home. Walk around while taking a phone call, march in place while watching your favorite show on televison, set a timer for 10 minutes and go up and down the stairs - the possibilities are endless!

I'm just too tired......

"I go to bed and wake up tired every darn day!" Quote by me, myself & moi! True story so I get it - but what if you convinced yourself that after a walk you would get a great nap/better night's sleep or even have more energy? We know that moving our body boosts oxygen circulation which in turn supports energy production so why not take advantage of this? Furthermore, walking in particular has been proven to significantly improve one's mood and can help relieve tension and anger. I live in the Midwest where winter is long, dark and cold and seasonal depression can set in. Walking even for 10 minutes outside definitely helps to lift my spirits. It's like a free cup of anti-d'espresso!

One of my favorite tricks is to wake up (tired), put on my walking clothes/shoes immediately, have coffee and a little nibble and out the door I go. The same principle has worked for me at the end of the day as well. I walk in the door, change and take a 30 minute walk before starting dinner. I promise you will have more energy and will begin to actually look forward to this becoming a part of your weekly routine (minus the making dinner bit).

I hate sweating.……

Sugar does melt when it gets wet but this excuse seems a bit silly. No person likes to feel sticky or smell stinky but if we start to view sweating as being beneficial to our health we can remove ourselves from the (arm) pit of embarrassment. Not only does sweating help your body cool down by regulating your body temperature, it helps to improve circulation and release endorphins in the brain that make us feel good as well. What a mood enhancer! I like to think of my sweat as just my fat crying so bring it on. But seriously, view a little bit of perspiration as being a really great way to reduce your stress while giving your mood a boost.

I hate exercising.…….

I have the most adorable neighbor who works remotely and when her young sons are home during the summer, she walks with them during her lunch hour and they throw a football back and forth. My point is you can have fun with this and even encourage your family members or friends to join in. What about catching up with a friend or loved one during a walk instead of going to a restaurant? Don't get me wrong, I love a good dinner out with some bubbly but honestly, my best chats with my husband or one of our three daughters happen during our walks where we can focus on one another without life's daily distractions.

You could also play the reward game to give yourself a boost of motivation. For example, if you take three walks during your week, you could reward yourself with a nice night out with family or friends. Keep yourself accountable by telling them about your new healthy habits and ask them for some extra encouragement and support.

Conversely, if you need a break from people and want to walk it alone, try listening to a good playlist on your phone or even a chilling true crime podcast. (I do recommend walking in a well lit, highly populated area when diving into the gripping world of crime during a walk if you know what I mean….)

Furthermore, we need to stop telling ourselves we hate exercising as our thoughts will manifest a negative reality. When we choose to let go of our limiting beliefs and feelings towards moving our body, we will achieve positive results. Of course we will still need to put in some work but how about we try telling ourselves we LOVE the way we feel after a walk. Or before we walk, we can feel grateful for the time we have to focus on ourselves or even for the legs we have to take us forward. It can be as simple as that. Your positive mind shift will eventually trickle down into your everyday life and I guarantee you will even start hearing people comment on how good you look from the inside and out - what motivation that will be!

I am too embarrassed to put myself out there…..

We tend to avoid situations that make us feel uncomfortable - we are only human. It is totally normal to compare ourselves to others when moving our body but this practice can have a detrimental impact on our emotional well being. The best advice I can give is to tell you that comparing yourself to anyone else will rob you of a joyful existence. Do you ever notice how you feel after watching someone on TV or on social media who seemingly has it all? We start to feel inadequate and a little depressed as we focus on what we don't personally have or do.

Keep in mind that everyone has started from somewhere and most likely have had the same feelings that you may be experiencing. You can go at your own pace and eventually build up the confidence to take on even more. Be kind to yourself and celebrate the small wins. Acknowledge every success you have had whether that is simply reading this book and wanting to make a change or even putting on those walking shoes when you simply didn't feel like it.

I could go on and on with all of the excuses I have heard. From it's too hot, too cold, too expensive to I'm too pretty to sweat (love that one) or I don't have the proper attire but deep down we all know excuses come from the fear of failure. We use excuses to stay in our comfort zone and to hide certain truths about ourselves. Old habits die hard and taking the first step towards change can be challenging but remember you are probably your biggest obstacle. Start by setting simple and small goals that are realistic and achievable. For just a few minutes a day, a few times a week, make yourself a priority and watch how your life will get better in all aspects.

4

Be Like Earl! How to love to walk like a dog…..

Let's expand the discussion on how to retrain your brain to actually like/love walking. My oldest daughter adopted Earl from the Humane Society a year ago and like most dogs, Earl loves to go on walks. Besides being super adorable, Earl tends to get a tad bored with toys easily and finds himself getting into some puppy mischief. Let's just say, putting shoes away when Earl's around is a must. Earl did get me thinking the other day as he excitedly brought me his leash when I mentioned going on a walk with him. What do dogs love about taking a walk?

The most obvious answer is the physical aspect. Dogs love to be active to release happy hormones - sound familiar? When we are done walking Earl (or Early Bird as we call him), he runs in the house, drinks feverishly out of his water bowl and flops down on his pillow for a nice long nap. Earl rewards himself the same darn way every darn time we finish our walk. Again, does this scenario ring any bells?

Have you ever taken a dog on a walk or even just observed one in action?

12

The amount of sniffing and exploring that occurs is just too funny. Dogs love to explore their surroundings on a walk which is great for their mental stimulation as well. Like Earl, there are times I just unplug from everything and walk in silence taking in the sights and smells around me (It's super fun walking in the country when farmers are spreading manure but you get my drift). This practice really grounds me and enables me to concentrate on my thoughts and emotions without being distracted.

If boredom is an issue for you similar to when Earl starts venturing into the bathroom wastebasket, try switching things up. Often, my husband and I will drive to different neighborhoods for our walks for a change of scenery and to explore - just like Earl. Change up your route if you find yourself getting bored and pay attention to how you feel afterwards. You could even try discovering five new things you have never noticed before on your daily walk.

Do you ever wonder why dogs greet each other with a butt sniff? (Can you imagine where I am going with this?) Well since this is a book about walking down the weight, we won't dive too deep into this topic but most dogs love to be social and sniffing their buddies' derrieres is a way for them to get a brief biography of their new furry pals. Now I am not suggesting we start sniffing other people's bums, but imagine if you used your walk as a way to connect with others socially. Think about joining a walking group or even a social media group that loves to talk about walking while keeping one another accountable. I have been known to even catch up with out of town family members on a call during my walk which really makes the time fly and the experience so much more enjoyable.

Even if you are the most introverted person in the world, can you imagine if you never saw another human being? (Wait, don't honestly answer that). Walks are a great way to smile at a stranger or even bump into someone old or new for a little chat.

The moral of the story here is whether you are looking for a social connection or simply interested in finding more happiness and contentment in your life, you need to be more like Earl (minus the butt sniffing) and get excited about taking a walk

5

Can I really walk down the weight? Does a bear poop in the woods…..

By now, we know that moving our bodies can positively impact our emotional health but can walking actually help us lose weight? It's a well known fact that we need to burn more calories than we consume in order to lose weight and walking is the perfect low-intensity way to speed the process up a bit. Any increase in activity level will bring health benefits however there are a few things we can do to speed up the process of actually walking down the weight. First and foremost - JUST START! I want you to stick to this long-term so go slow if you are just beginning and do not beat yourself up if you miss a scheduled day. Life happens and you need to have patience with yourself and this process and there is always tomorrow.

Did I say schedule? Without overhauling your entire life, think about your daily routine and squeeze some YOU time in there. Even if you only have time for a 10 minute walk in the beginning, that's progress. Eventually, you will find more time and you will actually look forward to your scheduled walk - I promise!

Once you establish a routine that works for you, you will find a few minutes more each week to increase your walking time. Try setting a timer on your phone or using a walking app to track your steps. We have all heard of the popular fitness trend of getting our 10,000 steps in a day which equates to about 5 miles. Don't freak out if this sounds daunting. It can be a long-term goal that you set for yourself and can you imagine the day you hit that benchmark? Party!

Now when you become a complete bad arse with this new way of living, you can even start picking up your pace for small bouts of the time, walking with light hand weights, or even tackling some hills. Walk down the weight by walking uphill? Sounds like a good plan to me. All of these methods can be incorporated into your new routine as your body adjusts to moving more frequently which in turn will burn more calories.

Even the most motivated people will have days where they just really don't want to exercise so don't beat yourself up if you have these feelings. Instead, think about what motivated you to begin this new journey and visualize where you want to be. Shifting your mindset will help you adopt a more optimistic, "I can do it" mentality.

Not only is walking good for weight loss, it has countless other benefits as well. Contrary to what we may think, walking can stave off arthritis pain as we age. As we walk, our blood flow increases to tense or tight areas and helps to strengthen the muscles surrounding our joints. Walking can also keep your bones strong and healthy, reducing your risk for bone loss later in life. Further benefits include improving lung health, circulation and digestion as well as reducing your chance of falling by building strength, coordination and balance. You can even lower your risk of heart disease, stroke, colon cancer and diabetes. The bottom line is walking down the weight can truly help us live longer and healthier lives. And yes-bears do poop in the woods!

6

Proper walking techniques and the 3 P's….. (don't expect more bathroom humor)

Most of us don't give much thought to how we walk throughout the day but it is important to touch on the three P's here: Posture, Pinching the Penny and Prevention.

One of the best cues a fitness instructor can give depending on the movement is to keep your head up, your shoulders pulled down and back while looking forward. The same principles apply to your posture when walking. Imagine that you have a string attached to the top of your head gently pulling you up towards the ceiling or the sky. This technique helps you to stand taller and avoid slouching or leaning forward during your walk. Proper spine alignment is crucial for maintaining good posture and preventing discomfort when walking. Try to just stand tall while keeping a neutral spine position. Again imagine elongating your spine by gently being lifted through the crown of your head. Think about how often we hunch over during our day whether it is sitting at the computer, staring at our phones, doing the dishes or even taking care of a loved one. Slouching or hunching puts stress on our back muscles so being mindful of this will not only help you when walking but throughout your daily tasks as well.

Once you have the proper head, shoulder and spine alignment we can now begin to pinch the penny. I clearly am aging myself here but it really is an oldie but goody! Imagine you have a penny between your butt cheeks and you need to squeeze your glutes extra hard to prevent the penny from falling out. How embarrassing would that be on your walk! Why the heck are we talking about money between our booty cheeks? Our glutes help to stabilize our hips, core and lower back muscles which are all very important muscles for improving posture and aid in the prevention of injuries. Oftentimes, our jobs or lifestyles require a fair amount of sitting throughout the day which can cause our glutes to be underused and weakened. By incorporating the pinch the penny method, we can begin to fire up those muscles.

Once the glutes are activated, we can begin to think about core engagement. Imagine you are about to be punched in the gut (wow what fun!) Your belly button would immediately be pulled in towards your spine as you brace for impact. Again, sounds awful but our core muscles play an important role when walking and help us move more easily by maintaining balance and stability. To summarize, we want to pay attention to keeping our glutes and core properly engaged during our walk and really throughout our day.

As we now know, walking offers up a host of benefits no matter what age you are. Not only will you be strengthening your body, you will be preventing future injuries as well. We often take our balance for granted but as we age we may experience a loss of muscle mass, flexibility and even worsening eyesight. Poor balance can lead to falls which can lead to serious health complications down the road. The good news is walking can help to improve your balance by strengthening your lower body, helping you to live independently longer and a happier injury free life.

Even though walking is basically free to all of us, I would recommend getting a pair of well fitted, cushioned, athletic shoes that provide good support. Walking paths and hiking trails can be so nurturing for many reasons, however you do have to be careful of uneven terrain or other obstacles like rocks, roots or branches that can cause ankle injuries. Walking on a sidewalk will most likely be your safest bet and don't forget to pay attention to the world around you. In other words, look both ways before you cross the street. If you choose to take a walk in the evening, reflective clothing can be a life saver.

Avoid blisters by wearing a good pair of socks that can wick away moisture and provide an extra cushioned barrier. If you do experience any unwanted foot, knee or other joint pain, I would advise you to slow down your activity and talk with your doctor.

7

Journal your progress! This is funny as you barely have found time for a walk…...

The idea of writing in a journal terrifies me for a few reasons. First and foremost, my left-handed penmanship resembles the work of a toddler using sidewalk chalk on a rainy day. Secondly, I often wonder who will find a little delight in reading about my deepest fears and insecurities. With that being said, I do understand the positive benefits of journal writing.

The first rule of thumb is that there are no rules. You can write about your goals, challenges, dreams, random useless thoughts (I have many), poems, even curse words. Sometimes it feels good to get it down on paper. You could even start a journal on your phone or computer if typing is easier. But why even bother? Countless studies show that journaling is a powerful way to boost our mental health by reducing our stress, anxiety and depression. In other words, journaling can make us happier. It can also foster a deeper sense of gratitude by noting even the little things in our day that make us smile.

What does this have to do with walking down the weight we carry? Our emotional and physical well being are definitely intertwined and when one takes a hit the other goes down too. Think about a time where you have been sick with the flu. Not only does your body feel like crap but your feelings of anxiety and sadness may kick up a notch as well. No fun! I am a firm believer that our health can vastly improve if our mind and body are in alignment.

The best journaling practice will be the one that works for you. You may even start with a "heck yes I walked today" check mark and that can be it for now. This is about you taking the small steps in your life today towards big changes for tomorrow.

8

Finally the end of this ramble…….

Your journey through the pages of this book mark just the beginning of transforming your life. Walking your weight down emerges not only as a physical activity but as a life changing experience for both your mind and body. Together we have explored the benefits of walking from both an emotional and physical health perspective. I hope you can begin to focus on your internal thoughts and feelings about incorporating walking into your weekly routine and truly reflect on what they mean. Are you telling yourself negative things? Remember, take the time to refocus your mind on the positive benefits of walking and you will give yourself the opportunity to grow and change in ways that were perhaps unimaginable before.

Just like Earl, YOU matter! Whenever you feel unmotivated I secretly would love you to chant this…… "Be Like Earl! Be Like Earl!" How much fun would you have walking down the street yelling this one out for the world to hear? Nothing makes us smile more than seeing a cute, happy, dog wagging his/her tail. Keep that in mind when you feel like you could use a ray of sunshine in your life and throw on those walking shoes.

Most importantly, ask yourself why you want this and where do you see yourself tomorrow? Are you hoping to reduce stress, enhance your mood or have stronger mental clarity? Perhaps you want to lower your blood pressure, reduce cholesterol levels or prevent the development of chronic diseases. Maybe your WHY is to simply be happier. Whatever your reason is, you can create the life you are worth living.

From a few playful attempts of humor in this book, my hope is that you find walking to be a practice that nourishes your body while shaping a healthier, happier and more connected life.

As we conclude this exploration together, your journey just begins. May this book be an inspirational and perhaps chucklesome companion to you as you begin your transformation. Cheers to finding a little more happiness and yes - a little bit of joy along the way.

I sincerely want to take the time to thank you for reading this book and for putting up with some of my comical or perhaps lame attempts to make you smile. If you found this book to be helpful, motivating or even a tad entertaining, I'd be very appreciative if you left an honest yet favorable (winky wink) review for the book on Amazon. All joking aside, my heartfelt thanks to you for taking the time for a quick and honest review as it truly contributes to the visibility of a book.

All the best - Joy

9

Resources

National Walking Month | Health assured. (n.d.). Health Assured. https://www.healthassured.org/blog/national-walking-month/#:~:text=Increased%20endorphin%20levels,and%20give%20feelings%20of%20wellbeing

Hannah. (2023a, July 27). *10 common excuses for not exercising– AND SOME SOLUTIONS!* The Heart Foundation. https://theheartfoundation.org/2022/05/12/10-common-excuses-for-not-exercising-and-some-solutions/

.Exercise and stress: Get moving to manage stress. (2022, August 3). Mayo Clinic. https://www.mayoclinic.org/healthy-lifestyle/stress-management/in-depth/exercise-and-stress/art-20044469#:~:text=Physical%20activity%20may%20help%20bump,contribute%20to%20this%20same%20feeling.

The Kennel Club. (n.d.). *5 reasons your dog loves going for a walk | Kennel Club Insurance.* https://www.kcinsurance.co.uk/guides-and-advice/5-reasons-your-dog-loves-going-for-a-walk/

Trust. (n.d.). *How to improve your posture when standing and walking*. MS Trust. https://mstrust.org.uk/a-z/understanding-and-improving-your-posture/tips-how-optimise-your-posture-standing-and-walking

www.ingramcontent.com/pod-product-compliance
Lightning Source LLC
Chambersburg PA
CBHW060905260726
48661CB00008B/3474